**I've Got Cancer of the Ar*ehole
I've Got Cancer of the Knob**

Written by Clive Bennett

Illustrations by Dan Prange

Other books by this author:

The Manners and Protocol of Drinking in British Pubs
Summer of the Pearl
The Blind Iranian Long Jumper
The Wand and the Tower

Me and prostate cancer go a few rounds.

An informative, if somewhat irreverent account of my encounter with prostate cancer.

The title is taken from a song by Peter Cook and Dudley Moore AKA Derek and Clive. Not only does it describe the region of the cancer perfectly but also men who remember the song are today in the age bracket of meeting the bastard face to face (or finger to prostate if you are going to be pedantic about it).

1 in 8 men will be diagnosed with prostate cancer in their lifetime. That's way too many. It should be a nice round number like ZERO!!!

My experience of cancer went something like this...

Mum called to tell me that Dad has got to have some tests for suspected Prostate Cancer.

Knowing very little about it, I research 'Prostate Cancer' in Google and end up on the Prostate Cancer UK website. I spent hours in the site just reading facts and stories and getting familiar with the worst case scenario (my own coping mechanism).

Armed with a bit more knowledge I get on with life and deal with only the facts, of which we have none right now.

Call comes from Mum a few days later.
"You're Dad has Cancer. Now it's OK because..."

She too had done her research. As she was clearly putting a brave face on it all for mine and my brother and sister's benefit.

The C-word didn't arrive in my ears with any less impact though. For anyone that has had cancer touch their lives in any way will know that the word carries more fear than the facts do.

My dad then went through more tests, an operation to remove his prostate and ultimately take control of the situation and survive the cruelness that is Cancer. An absolute hero.

I then read this book written by Clive Bennett. With such a direct and honest approach about his experience with Cancer, it made me feel so much better about my dad's situation. The way he handles the 'every day' with honesty and a big slab of comedy helps make it easy for me to understand other ways of dealing with a relative with Cancer other than fear.

Most of all this book makes me proud. Because Clive Bennett is my father. That was his (and our) experience, and had it not been for the speed and excellence of the NHS, the comprehensive support and information from Prostate Cancer UK and my dad's incomparable sense of humour, then I think we all would have handled this situation very differently.

Get support, deal only with fact and be strong for each other.

—Ben Bennett

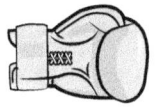 # Round 1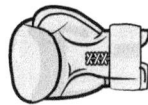

I thought of writing this book during the night after my operation to remove my prostate gland. The ward was noisy with nurses checking on patients, men were farting and snoring and I think I was a little bit high still after the anaesthetic. So here goes.

So, what is prostate cancer?

Prostate cancer is a thug and a bully, a real piece of shit. Like any other bully, if you leave it to continue its work it will ruin your life. We have to stand up to it together. Let people know about it, share your knowledge of it. The mystery of prostate cancer, or cancer generally just seems to magnify its ability to take over our lives, instil fear. Do not give this bastard any more power than it already has.

Now saying that we should talk about it more does not come natural to your average bloke, i.e. me. Now I have had prostate cancer or maybe still have it as I write this. I want to warn other blokes to get tested, but up until I knew I had it I would much prefer to talk about the things that come normal to us, Football, barmaids, cars and in later life, pensions. Blokes don't get ill, if they do they tend not to admit it unlike the other lot, women. They chat about their symptoms and problems all the time. We just ask each how we are using one word…

"Alright?"

To which we always answer…

"Not too shabby thanks"
"Fair to middling"
"Yeah, you?" Or some other innocuous phrase.
It is never
"No, I have prostate cancer"

I actually felt alright with Prostate cancer, I had no symptoms apart from weeing a few times in the night, but I thought that was sort of normal.

I am a beer drinker, so I know all about the number of times you piss in relation to drinking. If you are on a bit of a session I would last about three pints before I would have to break the seal and then piss probably every pint. I have never related the amount of times I used the gents to this bastard disease.

I seem to have digressed already. Back to the original question: What is prostate cancer?

Prostate cancer begins when normal semen-secreting prostate gland cells mutate into cancer cells. There is a theory that the more you ejaculate the less risk there is of you getting this disease. You can remind your other half of this when you come home drunk and smelling of kebab on a Friday night out with the lads.

The cancer cells may eventually form into a tumour which could visit other nearby organs and go on a bit of a beano (lads day out) around the body. On the other hand, there are cancers that are happy to stay at home, on their own and don't want to go out with their mates. For these lazy buggers the doctor will just keep an eye on you and you may never have to have surgery.

End of round 1: even on points.

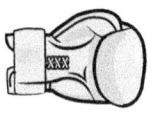 **Round 2**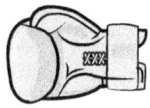

My story started with a blood test. A fella at work was chatting about his illnesses and reading between the lines I assumed he had some sort of prostate problem. He never mentioned the word cancer. I rarely do and I personally think its rude to do so.

Over the years, the word cancer has been synonymous with death. My wife calls it the 'old hurry up' on the account that if you got cancer of any form it would hurry you up to your final resting place be it heaven, hell or if you are a Buddhist, back here. So, by mentioning this word to someone, you are putting pressure on that person to come up with a relative response. This could range between "sorry to hear that" to "how long have you got". So, unless you go for the big sympathy vote which is more about you than anything else, then I'd use another word.

Mind you, I was telling one of my sons about my diagnosis and he did not get the fact that it was cancer until he chatted to his brother.

"Dad's pretty positive about all his problems, so why should I be concerned" were his words during his chat with his brother. The word cancer changed his viewpoint.

There is the alternative view of course. This is not to give the word any power and to mention it all the time. I am not quite sure about the latter, but it's your choice.

Anyway, the blood test. I went to my local doctor's surgery for a regular well man's clinic check-up and while there I asked to be tested for prostate cancer.

"Oh, we don't do a PSA test on this check-up it is too expensive" came the reply.

'PSA', I shall remember that.

The nurse continued with the usual tests, blood pressure, weight etc. and sent me on my way. I put it in my mind to call the doctor the arrange for a PSA test sometime in the future.

It was not a week later that I was in a hotel, training some students when in another room some surgical-type beds were being set up.

"What are you up to today?" I asked one of the ladies. She was in a type of nurse's uniform and having a smoke outside,

"Private health screening, whatever anyone wants we can usually test for."

"Can you do a PSA test for me?"

"Yes, we can do that."

"How much?"

"About forty quid" she said.

"Can you fit me in today?"

"How about now?"

"Lead the way" said I.

A little drop of blood and forty-odd quid down later, I was back with my class.

An official looking A4 brown envelope arrived about a week or so later containing a letter saying that my PSA test reading was 11.6 and I should go to my doctor.

11.6 what? I looked it up 'Prostate-specific antigen' I read a bit about it, and the number I had was well over the normal reading. Just to let you know that high PSA is not a definite diagnosis for prostate cancer and can just as well indicate other prostate problems.

As advised by my letter, I booked an appointment to see

a doctor, with the idea in my head that the next step would be the finger! I had to wait about a week. On the day of the appointment I was ushered into an office and sat in front of a small female doctor. Her face fell about two foot when I showed her the results and mentioned the word prostate.

There was no way on god's little earth was she happy about putting her finger up my bum.

"I think we shall need another blood test for clarification" she said.

I was keen to get on with the diagnosis and said as much. She was not going to be shifted. A blood test appointment was made and an appointment with a male doctor after that.

It is the day of my first rectal exam. I had been making jokes about it for the last few days. I had comments such as:

"If you feel something up you bum and he has two hands on your shoulders, start to ask about his technique"

"Shake his hand so you can check the size of his fingers"

"Take a stick to bite on"

"I hope you don't enjoy it too much"

"Start to worry if he takes his watch off"

"Look at the length of his nails" etc. etc.

The Doctor was a big bloke with a lovely gentle way about him. I shook his hand and done a quick check. My eyes watered!

I refrained from an attempt at comedy at this point although it was quite tempting. The joke was going to be

"Are you going to use your ring finger?"

It sounded funny when I was still under the effects of anaesthetic the night after the operation. To be honest I still find it funny now, ring finger? Get it!?

"Drop your pants and trousers down a bit and lie on

your side facing the wall" he instructed.

Sod it, I have forgotten my stick to bite on!

He surprisingly didn't seem to go up that far, within two or three seconds he was out again. I have to tell you it was a strange and slightly uncomfortable experience. I thought for a moment I might even shit myself, but no. I can also share with you that I did NOT enjoy the finger.

"Well?" I ask.

"Some irregularities. I will refer you. Where would you like to go?"

"Guys please doctor."

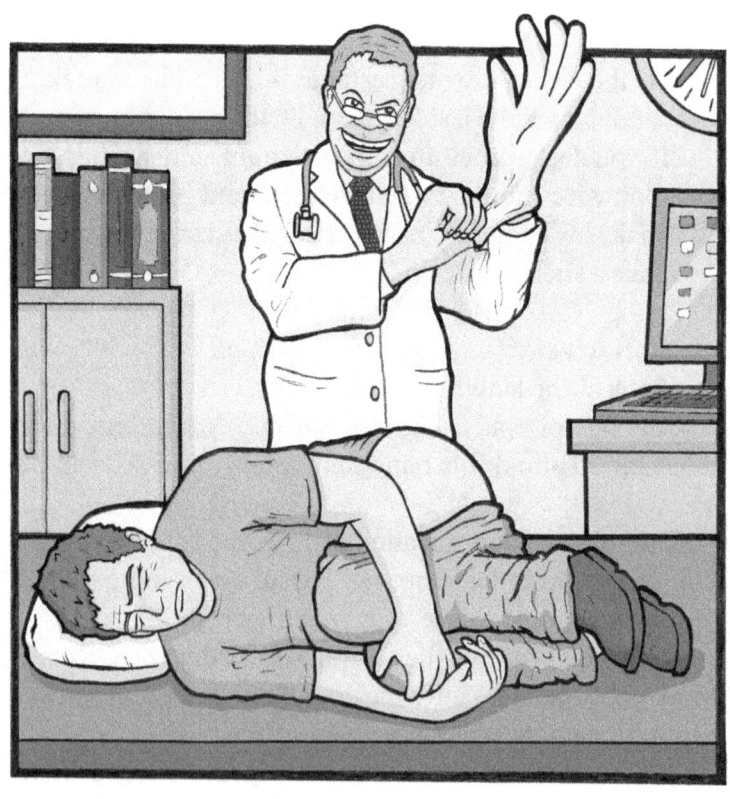

Luckily my wife had been all over the internet from the minute I received my PSA results in the post. She had researched procedures, professors and who was trying out what in all the latest techniques.

As I left that morning for my rectal examination she told me in no uncertain terms, "Tell them you want to go to Guys".

"Yes dear."

The first appointment came through quite quickly, within a couple of weeks if I remember correctly. It was an initial meeting with a consultant. This time it was to be a consultant's finger!

I had a letter telling me to go to the Urology department. Urology is all about problems with having a piss and the body parts that make up that process. I made the prostate cancer schoolboy error of having a slash before I checked in. For your information, you get the opportunity to piss in a pot nigh on every time you go to an appointment. The pot already has my name on it and a barcode. I am well used to being a number but I don't think I have been a barcode before.

I sat and drank a lot of water. In the toilets, they had a small cupboard to put your pot in so you don't have to carry it around anywhere. More blood was taken and eventually the finger. It is a well-run department at Guys and although there will be times where you have to wait, there are always a lot of similar aged men to talk to.

The consultant did not give out any declarations of cancers or tumours. Although he also muttered something about irregularities.

I am still hoping at this stage that it could be just an enlarged prostate, but cancer was at the back of my mind somewhere.

What he did say was that the next thing I needed was a scan in the nuclear medicine department. NUCLEAR medicine? WHAT!? Are they going to shove an isotope up my bum? Nuclear medicine, so I found out, is "radiology done inside out" because it records radiation emitting from within the body rather than radiation that is generated by external sources like X-rays. PHEW!

They could not squeeze me in for a scan that day so another appointment was made and off home I went.

The scan the following week was just a bit of laying still and doing nothing while the machine hums and chugs over your pelvic area. It is certainly the easiest part of the whole process.

"What did you see?" I ask the nurse, knowing that should could not tell me anything.

"Your doctor will meet with you and discuss any findings"

That meeting came quite quickly. The following week in fact.

"There is something we would like to take a further look at" said the doctor, "we will need to take a biopsy".

Now I know a biopsy is collecting a little, or several little bits of tissue to test.

"We have a new method that we are teaching here at Guys, would you mind if some other doctors were in the room at the time we take your biopsies?"

"Not at all" say I the eternal showman, talking before knowing the facts.

"I'll tell you a bit about it first, we don't put you to sleep but give you a local anaesthetic in the perineum."

"And where is my perineum?" I ask with trepidation.

"It is the piece of skin between your scrotum and your anus."

I am sure my Adam's apple went into overdrive.

"We then insert another needle which takes the samples. There will also be a camera up your back passage to guide us. We have developed a special chair for the procedure so your legs will be held in stirrups to give us good access to your perineum. The nurse will have chat with you and give you some information about it. Do you have any questions?"

"I am in your good hands doctor, let's just get it done."

The specialist male nurse, Jonah, was superb. I met with him on several occasions at Guys and he was always positive and knowledgeable. I went off that day with the first of many brown envelopes filled with information.

Also at Guys there are blokes called Volunteers. They have gone through the process of having prostate surgery and are now there to chat to and glean information from. Some were serious but others were quite light hearted and you can have a bit of a laugh with them.

It is best if you have a good sense of humour when you get prostate cancer. It helps a lot to laugh together.

Biopsy day was within a couple of weeks. As I arrived in the Urology ward a few 'suits' were wandering around being looked after by the hospital staff. I assumed these were doctors who are to be trained on this new technique. I had my blood pressure and a few other bits done before I went on stage. To my disappointment there is no stage or amphitheatre. It is just a treatment room with the doctor doing the biopsy, an American doctor doing a guided tour of my insides and two of the suits looking on. A lovely nurse was on hand to prepare me.

"Trousers and pants off, leave your socks on if you want to."

I think I left my polo shirt on and adorned a hospital gown.

You are asked all the time your name and date of birth, and I mean all the time. It is a good thing, although some people were getting the hump with it over the weeks of treatment. It is only to make sure that they have the right patient on the bed, so go along with it without complaint.

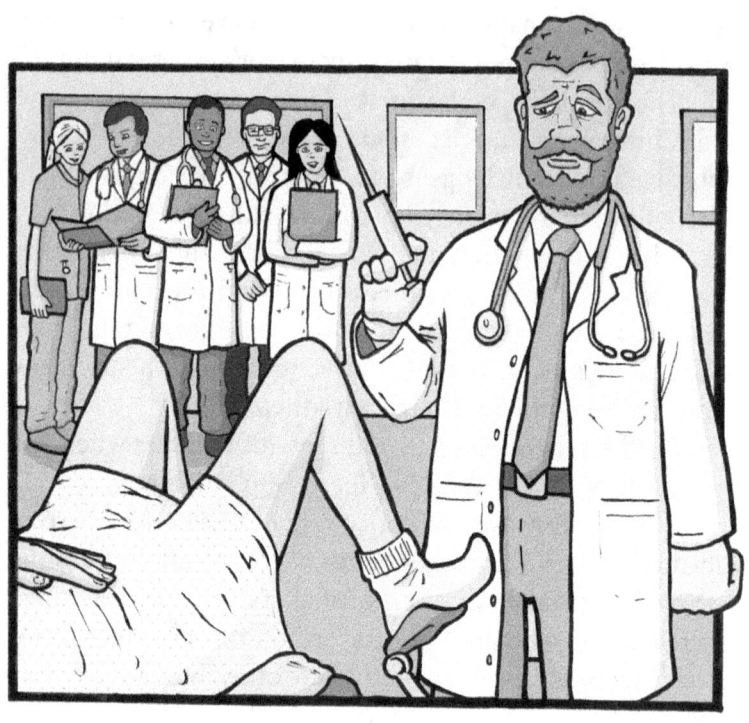

The legs were put in the stirrups. The lovely nurse has a large surgical pad which she sticks the bottom edge just blow my scrotum.

"I am glad I had a shower this morning" I thought to myself.

"Put your bits under the pad and stick it to your tummy" the lovely nurse instructs.

I obviously do as I am told and all my bits are now tucked away out of sight.

The doctors start chatting amongst themselves, involving me a little with "Any worries or concerns?" and "The anaesthetic may be a little painful but it is quite quick."

At this point the lovely nurse is at my side with sheets of paper.

"We are surveying pain thresholds and I will be asking you to say or indicate to a point on this line as to what pain you are feeling from one to ten."

Pain! No one mentioned PAIN!!!

My perineum was wiped clean and my eyes watered as the doctor doing the procedure holds up the longest needle imaginable. I am now looking around for the horse who is going to receive that needle. No sign of a horse. Only me. I would be lying if I said the three or four anaesthetic injections were not painful. I pointed to the paper, seven or eight. It was short lived pain and the other tool which takes the biopsy just gave me some discomfort rather than pain.

The doctors chatted throughout the procedure and I tried to lighten the proceedings with offering one of the trainee doctors the offer of a selfie with perineum. He smiled but refused.

"If anyone want to film the procedure for reference or to put it on YouTube, I am more than happy to oblige" I offer.

No one took the offer up.

The lovely nurse tried to chat about this and that with me to take my mind off things. She did her best bless her but my mind was on other things.

The procedure was over soon enough and I was left with the nurse to get dressed, a small pad was over my perineum to mop up any residual blood from the puncture holes.

"Now take it easy when you get off the chair" she

advised. "You have had quite an invasive procedure."

In my mind I have just had a few needles stuck in me and I am ready for the off.

As I stood from the chair my head went a bit light. I sat down and slowly dressed myself.

"Now you can't go home until you have urinated and also been downstairs to the foyer and back again" the lovely nurse instructs.

I wander just outside the treatment room to have some water and sit for a while hoping that my head would return to normal. After about ten minutes I decide to go down to the canteen and have a sugary coffee and a bit of cake. In my mind, it was sugar I needed.

"Coffee please" I ask.

"Which one?"

Now this is why I hate with a vengeance, pretentious bloody coffee shops.

Mocha this and Espresso that, Americano, skinny whatnot, you can apparently get cold ones! Why?

I am an instant coffee sort of bloke. I am not feeling a hundred percent and have the need to sit down sometime soon.

"Milky coffee, Latte I think it's called."

I get this information from somewhere in my brain from waiting in airports with my wife.
There is no sign of cake so I settle for an egg sandwich.

All is going well when after a couple of sips of coffee and a bite of my sandwich I start to feel faint. Trying to get some blood into my brain I put my head as low as I can without drawing attention to myself. I look around for somewhere to be sick and also the quickest way out. I feel like shit!

I start to walk to get out of the building but get as far as a low wall at the canteen entrance. I am feeling hot, I take off my jacket. I sit on the wall feeling faint with hot and cold flushes. I put my head in my hands and breath. I either fainted or dozed off after about ten minutes because I awoke feeling not too bad. Surprisingly no one asked me if I was OK, on the other hand perhaps I should have asked for help. I make my way back up to the Urology Department and find Jonah.

"I think I am OK now, I am off home."

"You look a little pale, do you feel OK and have you had a wee?" he asked.

I told him what had happened in the canteen and that I had had a wee which had a bit of blood in it.

"The blood is normal it will stop in a few days, are you sure you are feeling OK now?"

"I am a lot better than I was, I will see you next time."

With that I am off back to London Bridge station. At home I spend the rest of the day in bed.

Although you get letters through the post for all your appointments you also get texts which I found very helpful. Another appointment to discuss all the findings came through on my phone.

I had the need to do the whole cancer thing on my own. My wife was more than insistent on coming, but for some reason I felt that this was my problem and I wanted to keep it from her as long as possible. I have asked myself why, but have not come up with a definitive answer. After all, we are all different.

End of round 2: prostate cancer ahead on points.

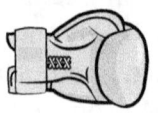 **Round 3**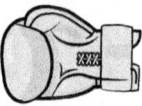

"You have cancer" said the doctor matter of factly in a side room "But it looks to be contained in the prostate."

With him was another person who I eventually assumed was some sort of social worker/psychologist but I never did find out.

"OK, so what happens now" I ask, matching his tone. I was not too surprised. My heart might have skipped half a beat but hey-ho let's get on with it.

I watched a Tom Hanks film recently 'bridge of spies' where one of the captured German spies replied when asked if he was worried "Will me worrying make any difference"

I have told myself those words going through the whole cancer process and it seems to help. I leave my wife to do the worrying.

The doctor chats about a thing called the Gleason score which groups the common grade cancer with the most aggressive type of cancer, the higher the cumulative score the more aggressive the cancer is. The marks are out of ten. Ten being all the cancer cells look likely to grow quickly. The lowest number that can be registered for cancer is six. Mine was seven.

The doctor then chats about options. Surgery to remove the whole prostate or radiotherapy were the main options. I believed I heard that if radiotherapy did not work then you cannot have it again, but if there is still a problem after prostate removal then radiotherapy is still an option.

"Surgery please" I say quite quickly.

"Do not decide now, go and have a chat with the specialist nurse and we will call you back in a week or so"

That night I did the hardest thing I have ever done in my life. I had to tell my wife I had cancer. We got through it, what other option is there?

I have had a chat with the wife about the possible loss of an erection after surgery which is common knowledge but both she and my daughter told me in no uncertain terms.

"Get the cancerous prostate out!"

A week or so later I am back. I tell the doctor that surgery to remove the prostate was my choice.

"A wise choice" he said.

"Now before we do the surgery I want you to go for a bone scan."

This is a new one on me!

"There is an outside chance that the cancer may have gone into the bone. If that is the case then the surgery will be quite different."

Contained cancer in the prostate I can handle, but bone cancer? I have to say I am a bit worried now. The spy in the Tom Hanks film can go fuck himself.

Another day, another scan, another hospital. The whole body this time at St Thomas'. The scan is similar to the one previously but a lot longer. You can keep your clothes on while the thing hums and scrolls over you.

Eventually the nurse comes in.

"I am just going to check with the doctor to see if he wants anything more specific scanned" she said.

She was soon back.

"Your knees, have you had any problems?"

"I have been a Plumber and heating engineer from the age of 15, a good time of that spent on my knees. I expect they are a little shot but I don't suffer with any pain from them."

"That's fine, that explains your knees. What about your jaw, bottom right hand side?"

I had a think.

"I had an abscess about three or four weeks ago, could that be it?"

"It could indeed. We will be in touch."

Another visit came through to see the consultant. The bone scan was clear. PHEW! I have only got prostate cancer, that is a result!

It is strange how your perspective changes when hearing different news.

The consultant starts chatting about robotic surgery. I have a view in my head of R2D2, C3PO and a couple of Daleks round the bed. It is actually five arms inserted through your belly which are controlled by the consultant with some kind of joy stick. It is the latest method of surgery apparently. I will be in hospital just the one night if all goes to plan.

"We would like you to attend a seminar which we run periodically. It tells you all about your stay with us and what to expect before and after the operation."

"OK, sounds good."

I go to another little room where I book my surgery date, I am getting a Professor this time, and get a date for the seminar.

The seminar was a week before the surgery. About 15 men are there, some with other halves in attendance. After the introductions, we are given instructions on how to improve our pelvic floor muscles as one valve which holds back our urine will be taken out and the pelvic floor muscle is now the only one which controls it. We practice clenching.

"Imagine you are trying not to fart in a lift or stopping halfway through a wee, that is how you find your pelvic floor muscle. Hold it for ten seconds and relax for ten seconds. Do that ten times, three times a day. "Also do some quick ones just holding and releasing for a second" we are told.

I have been told this now on more than one occasion. It helps stop the dribbling and MUST be done.

We are shown a film of the operation, it is clever, there is no doubt about that.

"Get fit before the operation" said the nurse.

Now I had stopped all forms of keeping fit as soon as I was diagnosed believing that the blood pumping round the body could grow and spread the cancer. WRONG! I am not the fittest bloke but not too fat either. I wish I had had this piece of information before though.

We are told that we would wake up after the operation in a recovery room and we will have a catheter. Now a catheter is a tube coming from your bladder through your penis and into a bag which is hanging on the bed. We will also awake to find a drain pipe from the stomach going into a bag and a drip feeding a cannula (permanent needle) which is fitted to the back of the hand. Sounds like so much fun!

There is a bit of chat about a couple of research projects that are being undertaken. It only involves giving a bit more blood and they take a sample of the tumour when it is removed. I sign up for that, why wouldn't I? Why wouldn't anyone? Every little helps, doesn't it.

A lot of chat about diet both food and liquids before and after the operation, which is well worth a listen.

What I have not told you so far is that I will be nearly upside down during the operation with my internal organs pushed out of the way and the belly filled with CO_2 to get plenty of access to the prostate. I remind myself to give the anaesthetist my phone to get a picture.

After the operation, we are expected to pass wind a lot. This is to get rid of the CO_2 in the body. Apparently, it can be very painful if it is not expelled, so fart away. I normally do not have problems in this area so I sit there and smile to myself.

"We will send you home with a blood thinning agent in the form of an injection. This will be administered by yourself or partner in the fatty bits of your body every day for twenty-eight days"

"Not looking forward to that one" I say to the bloke next to me.

"I haven't decided whether to have the operation yet" my neighbour said in the break.

We are now onto erectile dysfunction (lack of a hard on).

"Why is that, the cancer might spread and then that would be that" I ask him.

"I am not sure I want to live without me being able to do my duty" he replies, nodding to his penis.

It takes all sorts.

Apparently not everyone who has their prostate out loses their erection, you probably will not know for a while after the operation though. There is talk of injections and a tool (ErecAid) which sucks blood into your penis and then a band goes around the base of your penis to keep the blood in and an erection. The literature warns that the band should be in place for no longer than thirty minutes. There is a DVD given to us with all the information on this kit.

My television is visible to anyone who walks past my house, I think I may close the curtains while watching it. You may have seen the film The Full Monty, where Horse (Paul

Barber) is in a phone box with a similar piece of equipment. "What do I mean by it's not working, it's not working" he says to the equipment supplier. Hopefully yours will.

So, all on the erection front is not lost if you still need it. I believe this bit of kit is available on prescription. My wife asks why haven't I come home with one of these before.

Talk turns to constipation. We are getting information again on liquid levels and diet. It is apparently quite common to suffer with constipation after the operation. We will be sent home with a liquid called Lactulose which softens the stool. And if that does not work very well we will be taking a laxative.

There is loads of information at this seminar and also loads of paperwork to take home and study. Plenty of time for questions and answers to.

As my operation is the following week I have my pre-op done straight after the seminar which just involves a few tests to see if you are in a fit enough state to have the operation.

End of round 3: prostate cancer extends points lead.

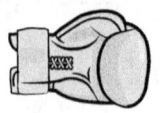 **Round 4**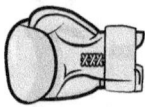

The day of the operation arrives. There has been no food past my lips since six the evening before and no drink since I have been out of bed. I have to go to the surgical admissions lounge (SAL) at 7am. I am gutted to be in so early as I have an old git's ticket which gives me free travel after 9.30. I am down a few bob already.

There is quite a lot of people waiting for various operations. We all carry little bags with dressing gown, slippers and wash bag. I am checked in and given another pot to wee in. There are two people with my surname on the board. I think 'what if the other person is having a hysterectomy, that would be very confusing for the surgeons if we got mixed up'

I am of course double if not triple checked to see that I am the one having a Prostatectomy.

I am taken to a room to get changed into some surgical pants, compression socks and gown. All my stuff is now in my bag and gets put under lock and key. A few more tests and chats and we are having a stroll to the anaesthetic room.

"We will be putting you out very shortly, we can offer you an injection in your lower back which will kill any pain below the waist. We find it very useful post op. Would you like it?"

"I would be daft not to, wouldn't I?"

An injection was given and a warm glow surged down my legs. I lay on the bed and a mask was placed over my mouth and nose.

"Just breath normally" was the last thing I remember.

I wake up in the recovery ward. I have heard stories of patients being sick when coming out of an anaesthetic but I was fine. After a few checks I am wheeled onto the main ward. I am in and out of sleep a lot. Checks are done on me regularly. After a couple of hours, I have a look below the covers. It is just as we were told, Catheter, drain from stomach, IV drip into the cannula on the back of my hand and oxygen sitting just inside my nostrils. I see my belly has been shaved too. I am encouraged to sip water and constantly asked about my pain. I am given pills to take, but I am a bit hazy on what they are for. I am frightened to move too far just in case I dislodge a tube or two.

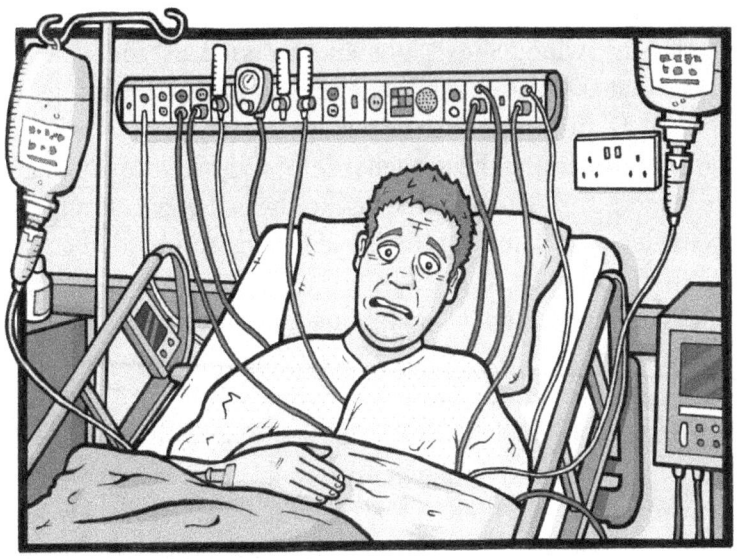

Night time comes around quickly, the lights go down but the nurses are still busy checking on me and the other patients.

At about midnight my stomach gives a rumble. "I hope that is not a poo fermenting" I think to myself, that could be very awkward. It is wind. Just as the nurse said in the seminar,

"We want you to pass wind after the operation"

I am passing wind like no tomorrow. Soon other inmates join me. I am reminded of the scene in the film Blazing Saddles where the cowboys are sitting round the campfire after having a meal of beans! Although the intensity and regularity of me passing wind slows down after about twelve hours it seems to carry on for a day or two.

The nurse said I am a good boy for passing wind and my insides must be working fine. I ask after her regularity of passing wind. She is not embarrassed as she clearly states that she passes wind on a regular basis. This brings a chuckle from the man in the bed next door.

In the morning the oxygen is removed, as is the stomach drain and drip. The bag attached to the catheter is strapped to my leg. The colour of the urine is dark and bloody. I am again encouraged to drink more. I give the wife a phone. She said the hospital had phoned her directly after the operation to say all was well. That was good.

I am allowed out of bed for some soft food. I opt for porridge, it is not too bad at all. I give myself a wash in the sink and go for a tentative walk. The catheter feels uncomfortable but there is no real pain. I feel tired and weak though. I return to bed for more sleep. After a bowl of soup for lunch I am feeling a lot better and venture to the toilet to empty my piss bag. There is a little valve on the bottom. It is quite simple. There is talk of me going home today.

I have a chat to some of the other lads on the ward. There is a wide cross section of society in here which tells me that absolutely anyone can get this bastard disease.

My surgeon pops in to say that all had gone to plan and they had removed a couple of lymph nodes just in case. He seems very positive. I am going home this very evening. My wife will come and collect me after the rush hour as we are going home by train.

"It may be easier by train as it is smoother than driving home" said one of the nurses. I am inclined to agree.

The operation wounds are re-dressed and I get gingerly dressed and have the last hospital meal.

I am given to take home, 28 injections, two types of pain killers, a liquid and pills to help my bowel movement, two staple removers, spare dressings, a couple of piss bags, a pot to put all the old injection needles in and two spare pairs of rather fetching white compression socks (I am wearing one pair). I am ready for the off.

With my wife, I take a very slow walk to the station. Within forty minutes I am back home.

End of round 4: cancer goes down in the fourth but gets up on the count of 9. The bastard is still ahead on points.

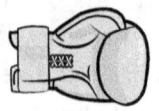 **Round 5**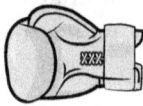

The first night getting into bed is hilarious. It wasn't at the time but looking back on it now, well!

I have to attach another tube and bag to the bottom of my existing one which I place in a bucket and undo the straps which are holding my existing bag to my leg. Bear in mind I am weak, sore and very tender everywhere. If my wife gets her hand anywhere near my stomach or penis I flinch. She is getting the hump with me already.

Eventually she manoeuvres me in a position where I am reasonably comfortable laying on my back. The tube is under my leg and going over the side of the bed into the other bag. Please remember to open the bottom valve on the top bag. I forgot to do this one night and I awoke with the inclination to have a wee. My top bag was full. I looked over the side of the bed and found the bottom one empty. I quickly put two and two together and found the valve to be shut. I blamed my wife the next day of course.

With the valve opened and the bladder emptied I am back to sleep. After each day I am getting stronger, more mobile and more self-sufficient.

Do not try and recover without help, you will need it.

I did not feel like doing too much in the first few days at home but I forced myself to walk about, but that is about it. I wish I had paid a bit more attention to keeping my penis clean as I had waited for the pain to ease off before I touched it. It had got a bit cheesy, so grin and bear the soreness while you pull back your foreskin and give it a wash or a wipe.

It seems to me that the piss bag fills up quicker when you lie down to sleep or just for a nap (I love a nap). So, check and empty your bag before you stretch out on the old settee.

I found the best way to do the daily injections is to ice the area you are going to inject for a minute or two both before and after you inject yourself. It is not at all painful with the needle going in but I felt some discomfort about a minute after the injection. The ice certainly helps. Read the instructions when injecting yourself. I met a bloke at the catheter-taking-out day who told me he had had a small stroke a couple of days before.

"Have you been doing your injections? They are supposed to help keep the blood thin" I ask.

"I could not get the hang of sticking them in sideways, it hurt too much" he replied.

"You don't put them in sideways mate" I said "they go in at 90 degrees; all you have to do is read the instructions!"

At this point another fella calls him a plonker for not taking them.

"What about the socks, have you been wearing them?" I ask.

"No, they were too tight."

One of the Volunteers came along at this point and tried to educate the man. I couldn't believe him!

The best way to get through the whole process is to do as you are told. There are plenty of people to contact if you are not sure. It is a major operation so don't rush back to work. Give your body time to heal. It will pay off in the long run.

Seven days after the operation I am on my way back to Guys to have my catheter out. I have been worrying about this a lot more than even the operation. There are a few other blokes up here waiting for the same thing. You can tell us apart. We are walking slightly funny, wearing loose trousers and now carrying a jug to piss in after the catheter is removed. You have to have passed a certain amount and have a nice straw colour wee before they let you home.

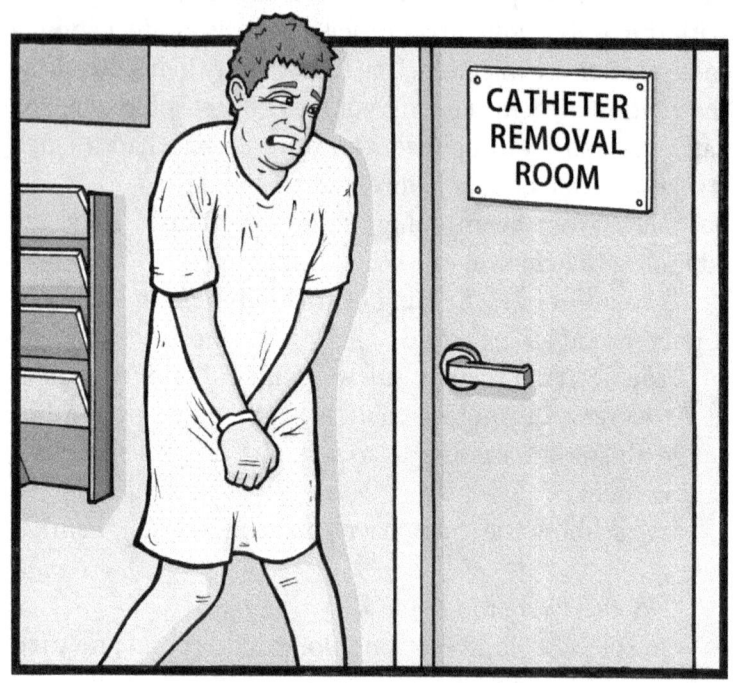

"Mr Bennett?" Came the call.

I laid on a bed with my pants and trousers around my ankles. I will tell you that any inhibitions you may have had about getting your tackle out in front of strangers albeit nurses or doctors has totally disappeared by this part of the process.

I tense up.

"Relax" said the young nurse, "I have done this before you know".

The catheter goes right up the penis and into the bladder where a small ball is blown up to hold it in place.

"Don't forget to let the ball down" I mention. The thought of that ball being pulled through my very tender bruised penis brings tears to my eyes. She gives me an old-fashioned look.

"I have done that Mr Bennett, now try and relax and take a deep breath."

On the word breath, she pulls out the catheter. I feel a mild tingle but that is all. I am more than happy.

After drinking about six cups of water, taking three wees into a jug and a bladder scan later I am sent off home with 2 packs of incontinence pads. I wear one home. Apparently, some poor sods have no control at all over their bladder and they piss everywhere. I think I am quite lucky as I can feel when I want to wee and can also stop it. There are a few dribbles (my new nickname amongst my mates) after I stop weeing and also when I get up from a chair or even laughing and coughing. Hence the pads. This apparently can take anything between a couple of days to a year to clear up. One of the volunteers always wears a pad when he goes out as he is still an occasional dribbler. His op was done several years ago. The answer to dribbling is to exercise your pelvic floor muscles and tighten them when sitting or getting up from a chair.

It is now seventeen days since the op, while writing this section and I am still dribbling although it does seem to be less than it was, so fingers crossed.

After about ten days I had an appointment with a continence nurse at our local hospital. We have a chat and a laugh and I am told I am doing very well. I am to expect a delivery of male continence pads the following week.

I have had a bit of a setback. I went to fill up my big wheelie bin with leaves and some bits of tree I had cut down before the operation. Once filled I pulled it round to the front of the house. WRONG. I now have a strain which manifests itself as a very tender left testicle and groin pain. I have done the cardinal sin of impatience. Please do not rush back to think you can do the things you could before. Give yourself plenty of time.

I phone up Guys for advice.

"As long as your testicle is not red or inflamed it sounds like a strain or sprain. Take pain killers if necessary and keep your scrotum supported, don't let them dangle"

I have my pad in my pants so I pull them up a bit tighter.

With the special tool the hospital gave me at my discharge, the staples in my five stomach openings came out yesterday, this was done by the nurse in my local surgery. She was very good and caring. It felt like getting pricked with a pin. There was no real pain as such. I was very brave and I did not cry. It is a relief to have them out. I seem to be healing up on the outside quite quickly.

Now I have realised that my penis is not as long as it used to be. This is because I have had a cut and shut. The normal order of things is the prostate is between the bladder (the organ that holds all the urine) and the urethra (the tube that takes all the urine to the end of the penis). So now with the prostate gone the urethra has to be sewn directly to the bladder, pulling it inside somewhat. So just a couple of tips when using the gents with a small(er) penis.

- Don't engage strangers in conversation
- Look ahead and inspect the plumbing. Do not glance to the side to inspect you neighbours cock
- Unless you have something particular to be proud of,

which we don't if having our prostate out, don't stand next to the sink or hand dryer.

I walked into a gent's toilet the other day and came across a four-urinal layout with a bloke at either end. The far gent was doing the correct thing, inspecting the chrome compression fittings. The nearer gent had this latest craze of having his belt and top button undone, waistband of his trousers and pants quite a way down and was pissing from quite a distance. As I approached the further available urinal, the nearer gent started swinging his thing about in gay abandon.

I believe I heard it thud on the porcelain a couple of times.

Jealous? Who me? Not really. I am happy the cancer was found and can live a bit longer.

It is four weeks to the day since my operation and I have booked myself in for work for the day.

This part of my job is not too physical and involves assessing gas fitters to see if they are safe to work in the industry.

I went for my first drive yesterday to get a feel for how I am doing. It seems fine. I am a bit nervous and have bought a spare incontinence pad to work with me. Everyone welcomes me back and the day goes without a hitch. I am a bit tired but, phew, a big hurdle done.

The next day I am more than lucky enough to be off to Tenerife for a week. The injections finished in the morning and it is really only the incontinence to be taken care of. We pack one big case which the misses will have to lug about as she has banned me from lifting anything. She looks awkward carrying it about and I feel really guilty. I get some looks which say "look at that lazy git getting his wife to do all the hard work" but what can you do?

We walk a fair bit in the warm climate and have good food in the sunshine. On the third day of the holiday I decide to leave out the incontinence pad while wearing my swimming trunks. It is strange that when I do not think about myself dribbling and it goes from my mind I am fine. It is when the dribbling comes back to mind that I seem to have a problem. Luckily the time I forget all about it is getting longer. I keep doing my pelvic floor exercise. I do 3 sets of 10 while clenching for 20 seconds now and follow that with 100x 1 second clenches. Progress I think.

While still in Tenerife and now four weeks and five days after the operation, I see that Spurs are playing Arsenal in the early game. I love watching football abroad and there is always someone else on their own who you can chat to. I give the bladder and the surgeons stitches a bit of a work out with a few pints of Dorada. I am then informed that England are playing Australia in rugby (Union) straight after. I can't go now, can I? So, I bath my lips with a few more pints. Unfortunately Spurs lost, but England won and I didn't piss myself, so not a bad day.

End of round 5: cancer still just ahead on points but I take the round.

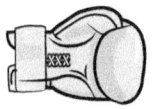 # Round 6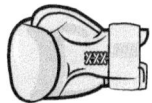

I have to tell you now that the wife has put a blanket ban on me writing anything about our sex life. It will also save my kids from some embarrassment as well. Suffice to say there has been some disappointments and some surprises. You will have to work out your own way of doing things.

The final blood test has been done up at Guys. Tomorrow I see the Professor for my results to ascertain whether the cancer has been eradicated. Cross your fingers for me.

It is not quite the result I wanted. PSA 0.21. Not bad I hear you say. I was, and the doctor was, expecting zero. His explanation was that the reading could be one of three things.

- Something benign
- A very small piece of cancerous tissue
- Cancer has spread

He made a point of telling me that the chances of the cancer spreading were very small as there were no signs of cancer in the lymph nodes that were removed along with the prostate. He chatted about radiotherapy in the event of cancer still hanging around. This of course would be determined by the results of blood tests which are to be taken in four weeks and then four weeks after that.

I am a bit down but what can you do.

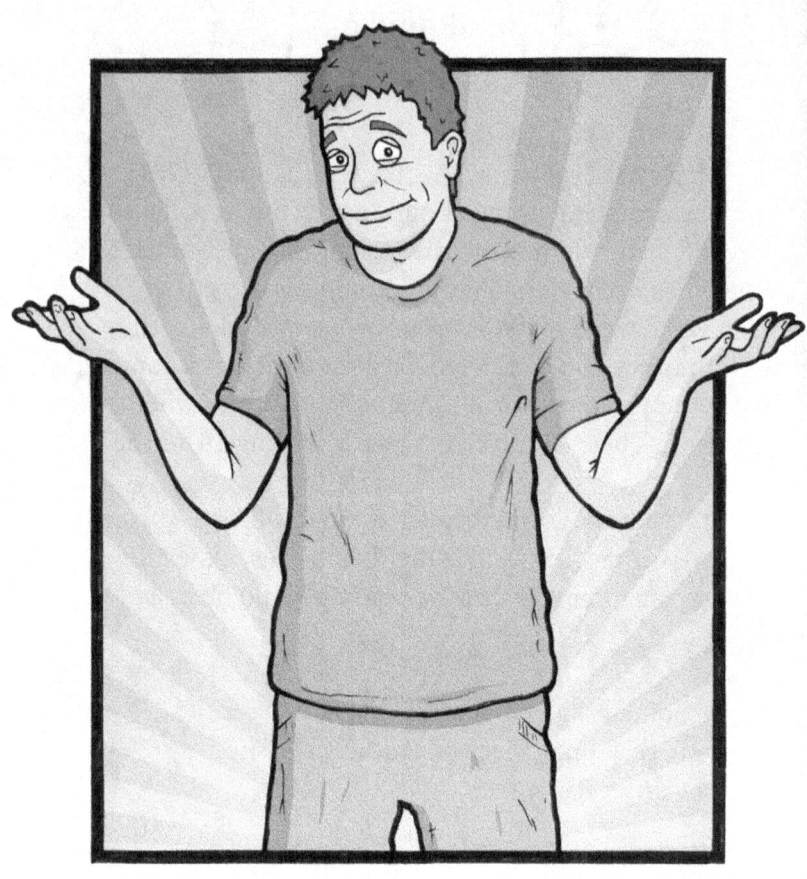

While I was at Guys I popped into the Prostate Cancer UK offices in Tooley Street to have a chat about this bit of scribbling that you are reading now. They are lovely committed people who make a nice cup of tea. Please support them if you can, every little helps.

At this point in time this book is going to print. If you would like to continue to follow my encounter with prostate cancer I have started a blog. You can find it at:

pearlyprostate.com

www.ingramcontent.com/pod-product-compliance
Lightning Source LLC
Chambersburg PA
CBHW070955220526
45471CB00007B/3041